Butterfly Girl

MY LUPUS JOURNEY

By: Aimee Ackell

ISBN-13: 978-1523774760

ISBN-10: 1523774762 (e-book)

DEDICATION

To my sister Ann, who lost her battle with Lupus, I will persevere and never settle for less than I can be, do, share and give in your honor.

Table of Contents

Acknowledgements

I would like to express my gratitude to the many people who have touched my life in some way, while I was on my Butterfly Girl, MY LUPUS JOURNEY and as it continues…

.

Chapter 1

A Little Bit About Me and A Little Bit About Lupus

"The beautiful thing about learning is that no one can take it away from you."

BB King

It was a hard decision to write my story. I wavered back and forth for many years. It is only until now, that I am comfortable in my own skin that I can tell my own story to help others heal themselves with having Lupus, or any illness/disease. I am a proud person, and it has always been tough for me to talk about my Lupus without being emotionally wrought. I felt embarrassed, ashamed and worthless about my diagnosis. I had no idea how to handle life, family, friends, work, personal relationships and myself. My life was turning upside down and I did not know what to do.

Now, I realize that I would not change anything in my life. This experience has taught me many things about myself, and it is all for the better. I now know and accept that I am a very special person. My journey has marked only one point on my timeline. I realize that I have a lot of life to live and I am going to live it to the fullest. I am a whole person who has come full circle through so many hard times along with the good times. I am a true survivor, and I hope that this book inspires you to become complete again, as a person.

My message to everyone who is struggling with an illness is to never give up on "you." You can truly accomplish anything you want to in your life. Do not allow doctors and/or people to label you. A label is something negative and it can affect you to not empower yourself. You have to find the right formula to heal yourself. Love yourself no matter what, or how bad it may seem. There is always light at the end of the tunnel. Love yourself unconditionally. You are the only one responsible for you. Everybody needs a little tough love to get them through a difficult time in their lives.

I've learned and I'm passing this on is when you are dealing with your illness, you are once far from yourself in that moment, but you shall go forward to be whatever you want to be once you decide to heal yourself.

Catherine Vidal inspired me to write my story to help others. I am fortunate to have her as my friend. I believe that the mind is a very powerful tool. It all depends on how you use it and develop it. The most important thing that I have learned is become who and what you want to be. It is a life long lesson that is a work in progress.

With these, few thoughts stated I hope that you enjoy the book. It can help anyone who is dealing with or without an illness. God bless and wishing you all the best. "May your life be what you want it to be and live it in truth. Look into the mirror and see your beautiful self, and the soul of your eyes. Your eyes tell your story. Make it a good one!"

"Smile, Smile More, and Cherish Yourself"

Aimee Ackell

What is Lupus?

"Lupus is an unpredictable and misunderstood disease in which the immune system is out of balance, causing damage to any organ system in the body. Symptoms of Lupus come and go, change over time, and often imitate other illnesses, making Lupus difficult to diagnose. Common symptoms include joint pain, skin rashes, overwhelming fatigue, and fevers that last for days or weeks."

"The exact cause of Lupus is unknown. However, Lupus is not contagious. While Lupus can strike anyone at any time, 90 percent of the people living with Lupus are females. Women of color are at an especially high risk. Lupus usually develops between ages 15 and 44. While Lupus can be disabling and fatal, the disease can be managed in most cases through aggressive medical treatment and lifestyle changes."

-Lupus Foundation of America-

Types of Lupus

Systemic Lupus Erythematosus

Systemic Lupus is the most common form of Lupus-it's what most people mean when they refer to "Lupus." Systemic Lupus can be mild or severe. Listed are some more serious complications involving major organ systems:

Inflammation of the kidneys-called Lupus nephritis-can affect the body's ability to filter waste from the blood, and cause severe damage. As a result, one might need dialysis or a kidney transplant.

An increase in blood pressure in the lungs-called pulmonary hypertension-can cause difficulty in breathing.

Inflammation of the nervous system and brain can cause memory problems, confusion, headaches, and strokes.

Inflammation in the brain's blood vessels can cause high fevers, seizures, and behavioral changes.

Hardening of the arteries or coronary artery disease-the buildup of deposits on coronary artery walls–can lead to a heart attack.

Cutaneous Lupus Erythematosus

This form of Lupus is limited to the skin. Although Cutaneous Lupus can cause many types of rashes and lesions (sores), the most common-called discoid rash-is raised, scaly and red, but not itchy. Areas of rash appear like disks or circles. Other rashes or sores may appear on the face, neck, or scalp (areas of the skin that are exposed to sunlight or florescent light), or in the mouth, nose or vagina. Hair loss and changes in the pigment or color of the skin are also symptoms of cutaneous Lupus.

Approximately 10 percent of people who have cutaneous Lupus will develop Systemic Lupus. However, it is likely that these people already had Systemic Lupus, with the skin rash as their main system.

Drug-induced Lupus Erythematosus

Drug-induced Lupus is a Lupus-like disease caused by certain prescription drugs. The symptoms of drug-induced Lupus are similar to those of Systemic Lupus, but it rarely affects major organs.

The drugs most commonly connected with drug-induced Lupus include:

Hydralazine-Treatment for high blood pressure or hypertension

Procainamide- Treatment for irregular heart rhythms

Isoniazid- Treatment for tuberculosis

Drug-induced Lupus is more common in men because they take these drugs more often; however, not everyone who takes these drugs will develop drug-induced Lupus. Lupus-like symptoms usually disappear once you stop the medications.

Neonatal Lupus

Neonatal Lupus is not a true form of Lupus. It is a rare condition that affects infants of women who have Lupus, which is caused by antibodies from the mother acting upon the infant in the womb. At birth, the infant may have a skin rash, liver problems, or low blood cell counts but these symptoms disappear completely after several months with no lasting effects. Some infants with Neonatal Lupus can also have a serious heart defect. With proper testing, physicians can now identify most at-risk mothers, and how the infant can receive treatment at or before birth.

Most infants of mothers with Lupus are entirely healthy.

All of this information is from the Lupus Foundation of America. If you would like more information about Lupus visit the Lupus Foundation of America website at www.lupus.org

Chapter 2

The Beginning of My Journey

"I will bear no affliction in telling my story."

Aimee Ackell

On the morning of February 6, 1996, I woke up in extreme pain. My knees felt like they were swollen the size of bowling balls. I could hardly move, but I had to move. I had no choice. It was my tenure year of teaching Fourth Grade at an Elementary School on Long Island. My legs and my hands were inflamed. I was in agony. I did not know what to do. What was going on with me? All these thoughts were running through my head and as I went to the hospital from school, I was not able to bear the pain anymore. I left school terrified. I thought I would lose my chance at tenure. My head was spinning. I was completely lost.

My hospital visit was ridiculous, a waste of time. I was there for hours, and left with no diagnosis. I went home with a prescription for Celebrex. I did not even know what Celebrex was or what its use was for my body. I was scared and confused. I did not know what was going on, but I remember thinking to myself that this was just a little bump in the road. Little did I know how deep, and dark this little bump in the road was going to turn my life upside down, in all ways. I was in for the ride of my life. Although, I did not have a clue as to what was going on or about to happen to me, I knew I could overcome any obstacle put in front of me. After all, I was strong, smart, pretty, successful, happy and healthy. How could anything happen to me?

After a few weeks passed, I was not feeling any better. I decided to see a rheumatologist. I had no choice because my sister, Ann Caroline Corredy, had Systemic Lupus Erythematous or another term for it is SLE Lupus. Sadly, she passed away from a combination of health complications and heart failure from her Lupus. The Lupus did not kill her. I believe it was the medications and the stress in her personal life. She was only thirty when she died. She was married, but not happily. My sister was a woman who spoke her mind. She was funny, smart and a hard worker. She loved life and loved people. Growing up, I use to call her "Annie Ba-nan-ie." She loved make-up, beauty products and clothes. She was the Make-up Queen. She worked in the fashion industry. She was eight years older than I was.

The irony is that my sister, Ann passed away at age of thirty with the same disease, SLE Lupus. It was unbelievable, I just kept saying to myself this is not happening to me! I could not believe it because I did not want to believe it. I remember sitting in the doctor's office in the examining room thinking to myself well maybe it's Lyme's disease, Rheumatoid Arthritis, anything, but not SLE Lupus? At that moment, I knew my life would never be the same and I was right.

Now that my first life was over, my second life begins and here is my story… I was scared, confused, and had so many questions. My life was crumbling before my eyes. I did not know what to think or do. What was going on with me? I thought I was always healthy. I was a gymnast growing up and seldom sick with a common cold or at least I thought and then I remembered that I had Mono in college. Everybody had Mono in college. I do not know if that triggered my Lupus, but I am sure it had something to do with it.

After college, I worked in NYC for a while; lost my sister to Lupus, six months later, my father died, and three months after my father's death my mom had double bypass heart surgery. After that tragic year in 1989, I married, attended Graduate School, and then started my teaching career.

My teaching career started while I was attending graduate school in 1990. I was fortunate enough to start working for Courtney Ross, the wife of the late Steve Ross, the CEO of Time Warner Inc. I was one of the original teachers who started with the school in East Hampton, New York, The Ross School. I was the Physical Education teacher. I loved my job. I had lots of fun and I was lucky enough to travel with my students to Europe, South America and The Galapagos Islands. I also taught a few children who came from some famous celebrity families. I really enjoyed teaching those girls. I taught at the Ross School from 1990-1993. I had a wonderful experience and a lifetime of special memories.

After teaching at the Ross School, I divorced and it was a very difficult time in my life. I was fortunate enough to teach at the East Hampton Elementary School for a multi-age class (grades first and second grade together).

As I taught that year, a few schools came to check out our program of multi-age and they liked what they saw. A couple of school districts called me to interview with them. As a result, I ended up teaching Fourth Grade at an Elementary school in Levittown, NY. Up until this point, I was completely healthy. I had no signs of any aliments or illness.

Now, I fast forward to 1996, the year had just started and in April, I would find out about receiving my tenure. Things were going smoothly. I was dating a prominent man from a lovely family. I was thirty years old and in the prime of my life. After all, I was young, pretty, smart, hard working and in love. I had dreams and plans for the future. However, life would throw me a curve ball or better yet pull the rug out from under my feet.

There I was, one day perfectly happy and the next day devastated. It was such a huge burden for anyone to handle. I thought to myself, after my first encounter with the doctor/s and hospital I can do this. I had no idea what my life was going to be like for the next twenty years.

The first year of my illness, I was in complete denial. I thought that I was invincible. I just kept on working and believing that nothing was wrong with me. I just kept getting sick. I was fatigued, my hands and knees constantly swollen, and my hair kept falling out. I was not myself. Many trips to the hospital, I had with high fevers and my body was disconnecting from my mind. I was not in harmony. I had never experienced this before; I kept on thinking and pushing myself to get better. I believed that I could do this. The bad news was that I was losing the battle. I did not know how to fight back.

One incident really stood out in my mind, which was with the doctor who had treated my sister Ann. I distinctively remember I had an appointment with him for a follow up visit. He came in and started to examine me, he looked at my hands, which was part of the normal exam. As he was looking at my hands, he proceeded to tell me that in ten years my hands would not be functioning properly, I would have cripple hands. My immediate reaction was disbelief, disgust, and horror all rolled up into one. I immediately got off the table and I was ranting and raving at him. I said, "How dare you tell me that from your mouth. I will be better than ever in ten years. Who do you think you are?" I am not able to write exactly what I told him because there are too many expletives that I used. I have dignity and grace. My mom followed me right out of his office. I do not think she was too happy. It was like a bad dream for her to hear those words since she just lost her other daughter to Lupus. In my mind, he was not human, and I never went back to him again.

The second year of having Lupus, I had a calamitous incident. I was at my boyfriend's house in Montauk eating lunch. I was sitting at the table, and he was standing faced away from me at the kitchen sink. He was asking me a question, and the next thing I remember is that I was answering him, and at the same time, I put my right hand up and then it was lights out Sally for me. I do not remember where I woke up in his house or at the Southampton Hospital. The next thing I knew, the doctor told me that I had a Grand mal seizure. I did not know what it was. I was scared shitless.

I talked to the doctors as to why this had happened to me. It was because my doctor had put me on a new medication called Plaquenil and I had a reaction to it. I had a spinal tap done at the hospital to confirm that this is what had happened to me. My neurologist told me that I was not able to drive for a full year. Well, that was a full blow to me. My emotions were wild. I was up, down and scattered. I needed help and inspiration. Unfortunately, my family had difficulty with my situation too. My mom was my pillar of strength throughout my whole journey.

I searched everywhere for help. I tried holistic methods and doctors. I was getting better, slowly but only for a little while. Teaching was out of the question and I was depressed. Now, I was on prednisone. It was not my drug of choice. Nevertheless, it was the only one keeping my body copacetic with my Lupus flares. It was becoming my best friend.

My life was becoming complicated. I was dealing with school issues, applying for disability, worried about my job security and what my future would hold for me. I realized that when you have everything taken away from you, you become very humble. I believe going through a traumatic life experience has really changed every aspect of my life. You really have to evaluate all aspects of yourself. Perception is everything.

While I was still not able to work, I was trying to figure out my health issues. I had conversations with both my doctors and my boyfriend's father. He was able to get me into the Mayo Clinic in Minnesota for a complete body evaluation. It was difficult back then about sixteen years ago. You had to know someone and my boyfriend's father was a prominent New York businessman. He also knew many prominent doctors in New York, which helped me get into the clinic. I was so thankful and blessed. The best part of this story is that I had access to have my very own jet fly me to Minnesota in the dead of the winter. Minnesota is unbelievably cold. Cold like an Icebox. When you go to the clinic, you live there. They have housing connected to the hospital. It is too cold to be walking around from building to building. All the staff and doctors are exceptional. I had such a wonderful experience. My exam was thorough literally from head to toe. Nothing goes unnoticed by these people. It is fantastic.

Once, I was checked in and examined, it was definitely confirmed that I had SLE Lupus. Whoopi! How excited was I, not. I was actually relieved that I had a proper diagnosis. I thought now, I could move forward with my life and try to deal with my medical issues. It actually gave me a sense of calm knowing exactly what was wrong with my body. I felt that I had a better handle on myself. It was all a positive experience. I loved the Mayo Clinic. I advise anyone who has a serious illness to go there and have a full body examination. They are excellent diagnosticians. For me, it was an awesome educational experience. I learned a lot about my body and many medical terms. I learned how to ask the right questions and speak to the doctors in a way that benefited me. I have learned in life, one must try to take the emotion out of a situation in order to make the right decision. It applies to everything.

After my period of denial, I went back to work for only a short time. I had to make a decision about work. The question raised to me by doctors was could I really work. I had been through so much at this point, and little did I know it was only the beginning of my journey. I came to the decision about working and then taking time off. I did this on and off for a while.

I decided to go and get some mental help and support by going to therapy. My experience with therapy was not a positive one. It just made me realize how depressing my life was and how my future would be for me. As you read the book, I will expand upon my "sessions" with therapy.

I think my family had a difficult time with my Lupus more than I did. After all, I had lost my sister and now it had afflicted me. Every time I would get sick, my family got upset. At first, I thought it was I, but it had nothing to do with me. However, for them it was history repeating itself. It was like having a bad nightmare repeatedly. I noticed this pattern. In the beginning, it really bothered me, but through therapy, I recognized that I was not the person they were upset with at all. They were upset at the whole situation. I learned that it was their plate, not mine. This was one of the positives; I walked away with from therapy.

My mom has always been there for me since the beginning of my journey. She has seen me through the good, the bad, and the ugly. We have become very close and our relationship is different than most. We have many difficulties, but we understand each other. I am truthful with her and she with me. I am fortunate to have her in my life. There were many times when my emotions were volatile from the medication. The medications over took me, both emotionally and physically. Emotionally, it was difficult. I would get upset very easily and physically my weight was a yo-yo. I went from extreme weight loss to gaining weight, overtime. My self-image should have been horrible. Nevertheless, I remember saying that "I always have to look good, no matter what" I always lived by that motto and still do. Your self-esteem and self-confidence are everything. You have to have it in order to do anything in your life. It does not matter if you have an illness or not. Believe in yourself.

At first, I can remember when I would be upset and depressed. I had a plan in my head and I would say, "I'm allowed only two days to have a pity party for myself." I believed it was a healthy way to let out my emotions. I would also try to keep up with some type of physical activity, but it was limited and so was I. I felt my life was closing down and spiraling out of control. It was difficult for me to deal with however, I always knew I had to keep moving forward and never give up. I thought to be positive even though I would have a lot of down moments.

It was time for me to start organizing the emotional and physical components of my life. I started to realize that I cannot be depressed, and I started taking care of myself. I decided to move onto the next phase of trying to deal with this "Lupus."

I started working hard again, and my personal life was about to have a difficult turn. I decided to leave a relationship of six years. I woke up one New Year's Day morning, turned to my partner, and said, "What's your decision about our relationship?" He knew exactly what I meant.

At that moment, based upon my Lupus diagnosis I decided to stand up for myself and ask, "Are you going to marry me?" For the last six years of my life, I have given every bit of myself. I cannot do this anymore. I cannot and will not. I am no longer for the taking. I am worth more than you can ever have in your life. I am! "Do you hear me?" The decision was painful. If you can believe it, it took him fifty-two days to call me. Well, I could not believe it. We tried talking things out, but nothing ever came of it.

I believe that he loved me, but he did not want the responsibility of marriage. I loved his family, especially his mom and dad. Unfortunately, they were upset over the situation as well. They were fantastic to me and taught me so many things about life. The one thing that I took away from them was how to treat people, be kind, give to others and try not to judge other people, sit back watch and listen. I also learned to listen when people talk to me. I can really learn a lot about them.

The best memories that I have from dating him were going cross-country twice by motorcycle and seeing the United States. I have to say that those trips were some of my best travels. I really enjoyed them. We had a wonderful time together. We journeyed and explored together, seeing amazing things and experiencing things that you would do once in a lifetime. I will always treasure those moments in my life. It was such a positive and happy time in my life.

To this day, I am still close with two of his sisters and one of his sister–in-laws. They are very special to me and will always be. They helped me out in a time in my life, when I desperately needed help and support. I will always be grateful to them for their kindness and understanding. The tremendous amount of motivation they gave me helped me for the journey that I was about to endear for the next 17 years. However, I have been on this journey for a total of twenty years.

I must say that in the beginning of my Lupus, it was a bag of mixed emotions along with a lot of unpredictability, about what was to come. I had good times and very bad times. The one way that I learned to cope with my emotions and incidents was to block out the bad, the ugly and the negativity. I learned a lot about medicine, my body, people, and doctors.

Chapter 3

Continuing My Journey

"Life isn't fair, but it's still good."

Regina Brett

I decided it is not necessary to describe everything that has happened to me during my illness. As you read about me, you will get my message. "I believe that sometimes opening the window a little does a lot more than opening it up all the way."

Realizing that I was in denial and accepting that I had SLE Lupus, I decided to take action to try to get back on track. I wanted to be "normal," but I knew that I would never be normal again. It made me very sad and depressed. Besides, the doctors had me so full of prednisone that both my body and mind were not my own. First, I had to learn how to deal with myself and then with others.

After I gave up my teaching job, and broke up with my boyfriend. I decided to take some time off for myself, which I needed. I decided to work for a while, and get back into a routine. I worked for a cable company. I was only there for six months. It was a complete disaster. Why, might you ask? It was because I was given the job based on who I knew, which was the owner and the owner's son of the company. It turned out to be a political nightmare for me. Due to my connections at work, the staff mistreated me. However, I was well qualified for the job and I enjoyed it very much. I worked in the capacity of an Educational Manager, who assisted in setting up schools to allow them free access to the Internet and access to the company's Educational website. It was an excellent resource for the school and I truly believed in it. It allowed me to do my job very well, which annoyed many of my associates. In other words, total jealousy.

By virtue of my situation, I decided to resign from my position. I was disappointed about this decision, but at the time, I had no other choice. I had no other options. I will not truly say what happened to me because I have too much respect for the person who tried to help me with my life, at a time when I really needed the help. Sometimes in life, you just have to suck it up and be humble. I knew that when one door closes another door would open for me.

I went through so much stress that I started to feel my body getting inflamed which was a bad thing for me, especially when that's what having Lupus is all about. Body inflammation has the ability to kill you. It almost killed me a few times, but I refused to let it take over me. I am a fighter who is relentless and believes in myself. I love life. I wanted to live my life. I just did not know how to find the right formula in order to get myself back to be "me."

As my Lupus progressed, I went through several battles of being hospitalized and had lots of testing. I was extremely sick for a while, and whenever I was ill, I would get depressed. Then I would dream, I wanted my life back, but I still had to put on a happy face. My mantra has been and will always be "You always have to look good, no matter what." The irony of my illness is, "you don't look sick, and you look perfectly fine." I could not stand it when people told me this, I might look fine, but you have no idea what is going on inside of my body. The major problem, I think with Lupus or other diseases that are not visible to the naked eye is you might not see signs of an illness, but that does not mean you're not ill. It is a terrible thing, especially for the person who has the illness. I always say and believe that if you do not walk in someone's shoes do not judge that person.

During my stays at the hospitals, I would always get high fevers of 103-105 degrees. Actually it was incredible, but not in a good way. I was always delirious. It would scare me. Nevertheless, I learned it was my body's way of telling me that something bad was going on inside of me usually an infection. It was very serious and I knew that. I knew that I wanted to get well, both mentally and physically I could not fight it. It just completely over took my body. Because of the high fevers, and given a high dosage of prednisone, I would usually lose about an average of ten pounds. My body weight would fluctuate wildly. I had three different sizes of clothes in my closet. However, I acclaim to have exemplary self-esteem and self-confidence to deal with my constant body changes. At the same time, as weak as I was I always tried to do some type of physical activity.

I always felt hopeful. I knew deep within my soul, I could kick this Lupus. I just did not know how to do it. I felt like a child learning how to write script. When you learn to write script, the key is to do it repeatedly until you get it right or perfect. I must honestly say that I am a perfectionist. When I do something, I just do not give it a hundred percent, I give it a hundred and ten percent. I have always been this way my entire life. There are pros and cons just like anything else.

The next thing, I decided to do was to teach privately for a Russian family. The family had one boy, and two girls. They were from Kazakhstan. It was my favorite job, and I loved it! I worked for them in total for about two and half years. I made good money, and most importantly, I really bonded with the children and the family. I taught them about American culture, etiquette, academics, policies and politics of the school system in the U.S.

They lived in Sand Point on a beautiful estate over looking the Long Island Sound. The family use to love to play soccer and entertained many diplomatic guests. I met some very interesting people working for them. They were kind to me and I was fortunate enough to learn about Russian culture. When I decided to leave it was a hard decision for me, but I knew that the kids were growing up quickly and soon they would be off to college.

Next, I went to graduate school for my second Master's Degree. I attended, C.W. Post College in Brookville, New York, which is now, LIU. I was in school for a year and then I had another flare up and hospitalization. This time it was bad because I had a mini-stroke. I had lost a lot of my short-term memory. However, that was not the worst of it, I was not able to drive for another year, and this was my second time of going through this episode. My neurologist was very careful with me. He is one of the best. He has his own practice and works at St. Francis Hospital in Roslyn, New York.

My life was hell and I had a hard time dealing with it. My mother did too, for she was the one who had to drive me everywhere and anywhere. You may be asking yourself, "How did I do it?" The answer is that I was intent on focusing and taking one day at a time. I was fortunate enough to have a few good friends. I believe that is all you need in life. I have many acquaintances but these people did not know me or better yet even know how to help me in a time of need.

Since, I was not driving, I was not able to work or go to school. It was very hard for me emotionally. I was always in a dilemma of what was I going to do with myself? I really did not know which made me have a lot of fear and anxiety about life. I would always think to myself; who is going to take care of me? Where am I going to get the money to live? Will I ever get married? I think the most important question was, Will I ever be healthy again? I wanted my health back more than anything. I learned that if you do not have your health, you do not have anything. You cannot do things that you want to do in your life. I believe when you have an illness it's a full time job of keeping yourself together. It is very stressful. Balance is the key. It was difficult for me to find my balance.

After abstaining from driving for a year, I went back to school. I worked in the Government and Documents department of the library and completed my second Master's (MSLIS), Master of Library Sciences. I decided not to take the library exam, but to work for a private investing banking firm. I got a job right out of school and started working in the city. I really liked doing business research. I worked with Thompson Business Applications, researching financial information for the Investment Firm. Sadly, one day in November only having been with the firm a few months, I became ill. I remember calling the doctor who was in the city. She recommended a drug called Keflex. I took it and I started to get a negative reaction to it. I stopped it immediately. I went home that night and I became seriously ill. I had a high fever became dehydrated, and very fatigued. It was the same reaction, which I had experienced before, and it was not fun. The following morning, I woke up and asked my mom to take me to the hospital. It was another hospital visit for me.

I had a fever for a solid week of 103-105 degrees. Each time I had a flare up it was my average temperature. Only this time, something was different. I was on an all time high of 100mg of prednisone. Again, I was delirious. I did not know a thing that was going on, but I remembered that I felt like I was dying. It was scary because I was highly medicated like never before. It felt like I was falling down into a well of deep water. I just kept falling and I was not able to hit bottom.

After a week of high temperatures, the doctor told my Mom that there was the possibility that they might lose me. They read me my last rights at my bedside. The doctors had to figure this out, as it was as puzzling to them as to me. They decided next to call in an Infectious Disease Doctor. It was the best thing that they could have done. It saved my life! I had a blood transfusion, which meant that I had all of my blood taken out of me. I remember the day clearly. It was a sunny day and the sun was streaming through my hospital window. My Mom was with me in the ICU room for the whole procedure. It was like an out of body experience, for me. They pumped out the old blood and pumped in the new blood. Luckily, it turned out well for me, within 24 hours, I felt like a new person. I felt "alive."

I was so happy and feeling better. I considered myself "blessed." I was grateful to the doctor. He was the best. It took me an extraordinary amount of time to recover from this Lupus flare. I had to work hard on getting myself back to a level where I could take care of myself. In addition, I had to rely a great deal on my Mom for her help. My life became a constant with Doctors' and Physical Therapy appointments. I was not able to work for a while. I thought to myself, not again, here we go another round of being very sick. It was getting to me both physically and mentally. Exhaustion from life had set in and my spirit was almost gone.

I learned that depression and stress are two detrimental factors to have in one's life. It does not matter if you have an illness or not. I decided that I needed to beat the odds against them concerning my depression and learn how to balance stress. My decision was to go to therapy, and the amount of time spent in and out was a total of three years. Therapy was, an up, and down experience for me. Emotionally, it took a toll on me. I had many issues to work out. The one positive thing, I received from therapy was if you do not ask you do not get. It was the absolute truth. My major issue was I was doing and trying to please everyone at the same time. It got me nowhere. I had to learn how to ask for what I wanted and needed in my life. It was a very powerful exercise, which taught me a lot.

The negative side of therapy was quite ugly. Each and every, session I had with the therapist was unpleasant. He would rip me apart bit by bit along with my family circumstances. He would tell me that I have no life to look forward to and did not give me any hope. He thought that I could not help myself get better. As I look back, I was in a funk and my mind was not clear. It was a time when I was on a lot of medication. It is hard when you are on medication that affects you both mentally and physically. You have a different outlook, and your personality changes. You are not the same person who you were before you got sick.

As time passed, I thought about my discussions with the therapist, and a bell went off in my head. I realized that this was not or should not be the correct form of therapy for me. I learned I was not going to take this nonsense from this individual anymore. I decided to end my relationship with this man. I ended it in a final therapy session with some choice words that I am not able to write down. To put it this way, it was not a pretty or an enjoyable scene for him. In my eyes, he deserved what he got. He was not a positive influence in my life. He was the opposite.

I learned that when I experience darkness in my life, I always try to look for an unseen benefit. During my dark therapy sessions, when he told me something negative it meant the opposite to me. I inspired myself to believe that I could do it. I just had to work smarter, not harder. I relied on myself. I knew that I was going to get there. It is not how you start; it is how you finish. You always want to be as positive as you can be and try to be a winner.

I realize that you can only learn from those who are willing to teach you to learn. It is important to have positive role models, teachers, and friends surrounding you in your life. I have learned that this has made all the difference in my life. Perception is everything. Whatever you perceive, you believe and that becomes your reality. I have done a lot of creative visualization with myself over the years. It has helped me tremendously to achieve my goals. It is essential that you set goals for yourself. You need to keep your eye on the pie.

Chapter 4

My Rollercoaster Ride

"Without a struggle, there can be no progress."

Fredrick Douglass

As I continued my journey, I was feeling melancholy and irrecoverable. My battle with Lupus was monumental and I needed to try to pick myself up and to move forward with my life. I decided to substitute teach I did not know what else I could conceivably do. I believe that you always go back to the thing you know best. In my case, it was teaching. I was not able to go back full time. I was too weak and frail, but I wanted to do something. I applied to work in one of the best school districts on Long Island. Actually, my mom was a teacher in that school district for many years, before she decided to retire after my father died. I remember going for the interview and thinking should I use my connections or not. I chose not to, and I got the position on my own merits. It made me feel good about myself. It was and still is important to me to achieve my goals and accomplish what I want in my life and never give up.

I continued to sub for a few years and then I had another misfortunate episode with my Lupus. This time it had to do with my kidneys. You know it is bad when your Lupus affects your kidneys. I had to have a kidney biopsy, which turned out to be a disaster! The information given to me is that the procedure would take a total of twenty minutes. Well, needless to say, I was on the operating table for four hours. I thought the doctors were a complete comedy act, like the "Three Stooges, Curly, Larry and Mo." I told them that too. I was in such pain and agony. The major problem they had was that they were unable to find my kidney (location) in the correct place for my biopsy. It is due to the fact, that I had an extra rib. They were not able to see properly to get to the area that needed to be biopsied. The results came back, and my diagnosis was Acute Renal Failure. I needed to see a specialist.

I decided to ask one of my most trusted doctors for a reference. The winning doctor was the best in the field of Nephrology, and in New York. I love this man. In my opinion, he is truly one of the best doctors, I have ever had. He came up with a plan for me and put me on Cellcept. He prescribed Cellcept, a kidney medication. In addition, there was a need to change my diet. The suggestion given to me was to eat nutritious foods that would benefit me and drink lots of water. The major problem that I was having was I was not drinking enough water. It is a simple thing to remember, drink water, but it is difficult to do. It took me a few years to get my kidneys back to normal, but I did it.

In the beginning, I was kept a close eye on along with many doctor's visits. My visits with the doctor decreased, as my kidney levels got better. Eventually, I got myself to a point where I would only have to visit him once a year to check on my kidneys. It was a lot of work, time and travel to go visit the doctor. His office was all the way up on the West Side Highway in New York. It was difficult for me at times, because my kidneys were bad. I just kept saying to myself, "I don't want to go on dialysis." I saw people who were on dialysis and it scared me to death. Kidney dialysis would have entailed the use of a special machine to filter harmful wastes, salt, and excess fluid from my blood. When you have this procedure, it restores the blood to a normal, healthy balance. Dialysis replaces many of the kidney's important functions.

As time passed, my kidneys were improving, as well as my mental and physical attitude. I learned that proper regiment of medication and a beneficial diet were key to having a harmonious balance for my Lupus. I was doing well for about a year and half. Then, I remember going to the rheumatologist for a regular scheduled appointment, which at the time was every six to eight weeks. The doctor came in and told me that my numbers were all down, like a sinking ship.

The tests that the doctor orders measure my Lupus activity and examine the following: red, white blood cell count, platelets, DNA levels and sediment rate. It means the following when you have Systemic Lupus Erythematosus; a complete blood test measures the number of red blood cells, white blood cells and platelets as well as the amount of hemoglobin, a protein in red blood cells. Results may indicate that you have anemia, which commonly occurs in Lupus. Having anemia can cause fatigue among Lupus patients. A low white blood cell or platelet count may occur in Lupus as well, and it indicates that you may be or you have it's an immunosuppressive therapy, corticosteroids such as prednisone, or the presence of a virus. The doctor usually tests for five different types of white blood cells. Each group of white blood cells plays a different role in the immune system response. It shows differences among the different types, and measures whether these cells are present in your body in normal proportions, revealing information about certain deficiencies in your immune system. Using myself as an example with my Lupus, and having been on prednisone for 18 years it lowered my lymphocyte count. "One's lymphocyte count is another name for white blood cells. They are one of the cells of the autoimmune system of the vertebrates. The cells protect the body from becoming infected by bacteria and viruses and also fight off bacterial and viral infections." MD-Health.com

The DNA is the anti-double stranded (anti-dsDNA). It is tested in patients to help diagnose, Lupus (Systemic Lupus Erthematosus) and to see if they show a positive result for antinuclear antibodies. These anti bodies are produced in a person's immune system and when it fails to distinguish between itself and nonself, it affects the nucleus of cells. This Anti-dsDNA specifically target the genetic material (DNA) found in the nucleus, causing organ and tissue damage. In my case, my symptoms were muscle pain, arthritis, red rashes on my face which resembled a butterfly across my nose and cheeks (malar rash), persistent fatigue, weakness, skin sensitivity, numbness/tingling in my hands/feet, inflammation damage to my organs and tissues, including my kidneys, lungs, heart, central nervous system, blood vessels, hair and weight loss. The sediment rate detects and monitors the amount of inflammation in the body.

After receiving the results, and having serious discussions with my physician, he decided to put me on Chemotherapy. I must tell you that I did not want to do it. I fought with him for many months. Once I made the decision to go ahead with the chemo, I had to have a Port put into my chest. The Port was necessary because chemo is toxic, and can damage both your skin and muscle tissue. They place it beneath the skin. A catheter connects the port to a vein. The port located under the skin has a septum through which drugs are flowing through you and blood samples can be drawn many times, usually with less discomfort and better than the typical needle stick. The results of having it were disastrous and dangerous. The chemo brought about change, but not the change I wanted.

I was fortunate enough to have my chemo administered to me at my home. It was a huge blessing. Each time, I would receive the chemo it took many hours, and I was completely exhausted. The nurses were always very good to me, and I endured the complete "hell" of it. At the time of my treatments, I had several of my friends visit me during this period. The one thing that sticks out in my mind about receiving the treatments was when the medicine initially entered into my port and flowing through my veins, it felt like my body was burning on the inside. It frightened me and made me uncomfortable. I hated the chemo treatments. I had a feeling the entire time that nothing good was happening to my body. There was change going on, but not any good change. It was destroying me.

The change that the chemo brought to me was both physically and mentally grueling. It was as if someone took a stamp from a stamp pad and marked me unfit for life. I had many physical changes to my body. I had all of my hair fall out, which I just absolutely loved. As a little girl, my mother would never let me have long hair, and as I grew older, I always kept my hair long. I coveted my hair. My hair was a sign to me of my power and strength. After losing all my hair, I would go to the hairdresser every three weeks and have him trim whatever little hair growth I had on my head. I tried to keep my dignity. It is very hard keeping your dignity when you feel ugly and powerless. I believe that you cannot understand these feelings until it happens to you personally. I am aware that people do not understand what you are going through unless they have walked down the same path as you. If they have a similar experience as you, then they are able to relate to what is happening to them in their life.

For two years, I was on Cytoxan one of the strongest Chemos, and I can honestly say it did zero for me. There was no explanation as to why I had to have this type of chemo. It gave me some permanent issues that I have to deal with for the rest of my life, which I did not know about or asked for them. Complaining gets you nowhere. I believe whatever God gives you, you have to deal with it and move forward and never look back. The permanent issues, I was given neuropathy in my feet, shingles in my right eye three times, not being able to have children, and the real kicker was that I went through menopause at age 40. I cannot tell you the layers of anger, and levels of pain that I went through to deal with each of these problems. I think that it is only natural to have felt sadness, anger, hurt, disappointment, depression and resentment.

Another change that I had endured with chemo was that I had severe third degree burns on my face. It was to say the least, horrifying to me both mentally and physically. Unfortunately, the doctor did not tell me about that being one of the side effects. I guess as in Lupus and with chemo, it affects each individual differently. I felt very defeated at this point in my treatment. I knew I could handle the loss of my hair, I knew it would grow back and not be permanent. However, my face was a different story. I had always had such beautiful skin, and I had always taken such good care of it. Not only that, but I was blessed with good genes too. I tried everything to cover up the redness all over my face. I went to specialists, medical beauty spas, and various department stores looking for something to cover my face. After many months of searching, I found a product put out by Clinique that provided me with coverage for my face, and it proved to be helpful. I was relieved and happy at the same time. It is because of that I was able to overcome my hurdles with chemo.

The chemo made me extremely sick and weak. I was always tired, and I felt that I had little normalcy left in my life. However, I kept saying to myself, "never give up, you're a fighter, a survivor and you can beat this." I struggled each day, but I knew that I wanted to move forward, and try to get better. I have always said, and believed that "no matter how bad it gets I have to feel pretty." I always tried to make myself feel pretty which lead me to believe that I could conquer "my Lupus."

After my chemo ended, I swear my body went quickly into a menopausal stage. I started with hot flashes and night sweats. I was a hot mess. Every night, I would have to change my P.J.s at least four times a night. It was grueling. I was lucky that I did not have a lot of heavy mood swings and the other symptoms that went along with menopause. I did not have a normal menopause. Chemotherapy caused me to have my menopause. I was so pissed off about it because no one told me about the menopausal changes that could happen to me. I was blind sided by this and I did not even think or know about saving my eggs for the future. Little did I know that I had no future of having a family? In all honesty, if I were stronger and healthier, I would have made better decisions about handling my body. Unfortunately for me at the time, I was too weak and emotionally distraught. I will tell you one thing that I learned from having gone through what I've gone through, don't treat your disease emotionally. You have to deal with it as if it were a business deal. If you think of it as business, you make better decisions about your health and the path that you want to take to achieve your goals. I think that you will become an all round winner, if you think of yourself first.

As they say in baseball, "Who's up next in the batting line up?" My feet were up next in the line up for one of the several side effects from the chemo. My nerve damage was resolute in my feet. My neuropathy came into play about six to nine months after my chemo was finished. I did not know what it was. The doctor told me that I had a chance of my neuropathy going away, but not completely. There was no guarantee. By the way, he was right. I was out of luck. My feet never got any better. I had foot massages weekly for three years. Sometimes it felt as if my feet were getting better, but they were not. My progress and prognosis was inconsistent, and I tried many other things to help relieve my foot pain. I am still trying with my feet. My neuropathy pain has always been a living hell for me. It is the best way to describe it.

Because of my neuropathy, I am not able to wear beautiful high-heeled shoes. Oh, did I have some gorgeous designer shoes. I have nice legs so when I was not able to wear sexy shoes anymore it made me feel depressed. Every woman loves shoes; especially high-heeled shoes, and the way they make you feel when you wear them. I have had to learn to compromise and go for comfort. I found that the only shoe that I am able to wear with a little heel is the wedge. It is comfortable and I am able to walk in them. However, when I try to wear high heels, the pain in my feet is unbearable. I just want to scream the whole time I am wearing them on my feet. The podiatrist advised me that I should wear a shoe that is sturdy and made well. I cannot wear anything flimsy and that does not have support. If I do, my feet end up throbbing in pain and it is not worth it. I have learned to wear only well-made shoes. It makes my life a lot easier.

The phrase "mind over matter" by Sir Charles Lyell, I believe to be true and very true for me. I tried so many different medications for my neuropathy. Unfortunately, they would only last for a certain amount of time, and then the pain would come back something fierce. I decided to do research on pain, and pain management. I came to my own conclusion that I would be able to try to control the amount of pain in my feet. I know it sounds like I am out of my mind. However, I beg to differ. I have found it better to take less medication and control my pain with brain imaging and positive thinking. It really works for me. I still have the pain in my feet; some days are better than other days. However, one needs to remember, "No pain, No gain." It is very true. I really try to block out the pain. I have done it for years. Yes, it is there, but I deal with it in my own way. I have decided that I want to live my life, and not have my life dictate the way I should live it. Spirituality has taken a huge role for me to build an understanding about healing my body. I would be lying to you if I said, "my feet don't bother me." However, the reality is that they do. I believe that my strength, power and determination have helped me deal with my neuropathy issues.

Chemo had broken down my immune system so maladroitly that I had shingles in my right eye three times. I had it over a three-year period, and it always seemed to happen to me during the month of June. I was in such dismay. Each time, I had it, I would wake up in the morning and rub my eyes because they were extremely itchy and at the same time in my right eye felt like there was a little rock in it. My eye would slowly become redder and redder. Eventually, when I went to the doctor, I was at the point of trying to scratch my eyes out. The good news was that I went to the doctor in the early stages and she had put me on Valtrex. Valtrex is a medication that treats herpes virus infections, including shingles (herpes zoster), cold scores and genital herpes in adults. Valtrex is an antiviral drug. It slows down the growth and spread of the herpes virus so that the body can fight off the infection. Valtrex will not cure herpes, but it can lessen the symptoms of the infection.

I also had to take eye drops, and drops with steroids to help me deal with my shingles. My shingles were a travesty. I had to endure excruciating pain, embarrassment, resentment and complete ugliness all rolled up into one. I am not even lying or exaggerating when I tell you I looked like the "Elephant Man." There are no words to describe my emotions about it. I really had to dig deep down inside myself and say, "I have to move on…if I don't, I will be beaten down." I was determined to win and not be a loser. Dealing with my illness was very much a mind game. I had to play both sides defensively and offensively. I was always on my guard, and with good reason, I always wanted to come out on top.

I remember going to my friend's Fourth of July party twice, and I had shingles. I was so determined to go that I put on my black quilted "Jackie O" Chanel type sunglasses, which were large enough to cover up my bulging disgusting eye and cover up as if nothing happened to me. I wore them for the entire party, and I never took them off, I did not care. The truth was that I felt ugly, sad, and just out of place. It was awkward. I resented the fact that I could not go somewhere and enjoy myself completely. I had to act as if nothing was wrong with me and my life was perfect. I must admit that I have always been a great actor and giving the perception that I am perfectly fine, but deep down, I am not. I believe that everyone has a story behind his or her eyes.

At this time, my mental state covered an array of emotions. I said to myself, "I can't believe this is happening to me. Haven't I been through enough? I can't take it anymore." I had suffered a great deal and had undergone so many physical changes. Enough was enough, but little did I know what was to come next for me with this disease. I learned that I had to take baby steps, and go day, by day in order to have a positive attitude and outlook. It is essential to try to be positive at all times.

Besides, the emotional side effects, I encountered a great deal of physical side effects from my shingles too. My vision had changed, and now I had scare tissue on my right cornea. My right eye seems to trail off sometimes when I am looking at someone. Often, someone will say to me "what are you looking at?" and in return I will say, "I have a problem with my eye because I had shingles in my right eye three times." Usually, people are taken back and do not know what to say. Most people do not even know what shingles are. I have to explain what it is and how you get it. I also have a scar on my forehead above my right eye. It looks like I have a hole in my head and I have had surgery done on it two times. However, you can still see it. Several dermatologists have told me that it is a difficult spot to fix properly unless I have plastic surgery. Doctor's do not like to preform plastic surgery on people who have Lupus. I think it is unfair and if I could have it, I would. I am convinced people in general are not knowledgeable when it comes to their bodies and their overall health.

I believe that this part of my journey was extremely draining on me physically, and I would not wish it on my worst enemy. I believe that my pain and suffering came to me in many different sizes and shapes. It has been cruel, heartbreaking, exhausting, and down right unfair. However, I have learned to become very humble and not to judge people. It is a big lesson that I have learned at a great cost with my own health.

Chapter 5

No Pain, No Gain

"We may encounter many defeats but we must not be defeated."

Maya Angelou

It was amazing to me, but I felt like the rain was never ending. My pain and suffering continued throughout my journey. I was limited in doing many things like work, socializing, physical activities and finding my health. I was in for the run of my life. After regrouping from the trauma that I had just been through, I slowly began having problems walking. I ignored the change happening to me in my body and just thought there was nothing wrong with me. I am famous for believing that my mind is stronger than my body. However, at this time I was not able to have my mind over come the pain, agony, depression and limiting as what my body could do.

First, it started with feeling as if I had two cement blocks on my feet. I would always shuffle my gait. I would say it went on for a solid two years. My quality of life suffered. Not only was I not able to walk, but forget about even trying to run. I was not able to play any sports, and I became very inactive which led me into a great depression. I was losing control over my ability to function as a normal person. I went to many specialists, and they would literally just feed me medications. They did not know any better, and I had to take it because I had no choice. I feel that doctors are so limited in helping individuals who suffer with intolerable pain. The type of pain that I had was severe, constant and never let up. I would go to work substitute teaching and people would constantly say what is the matter with your feet? In addition, my reply was I hurt my foot or I would say, I am just having some problems with my feet. I did not feel like telling anyone my business. I have always been a very private person. In truth, I did not like people judging me. I have felt that people were always judging me, and it bothered me tremendously. Feeling uncomfortable was an understatement.

As time went by, I continued working, and the pain in my feet was becoming excruciating. The rest of my body started to feel the reverberations from it. My legs started to have severe pain and inflammation and eventually it reached my hips. When that happened, I could no longer tolerate the agony. My body's demeanors both physically and mentally were at an all time low. I just kept seeing many rheumatologists and I was not getting any answers about why my body was in pain. I also had to see an orthopedic doctor in New York City, and it was not a pleasant visit. These doctors' visits took about a year of my time. It was frustrating and I ended up suffering terribly. My life had changed and was continuing to change forever.

I was bed ridden. It had gotten so bad that I was not even able to bend my hips in order to sit down and go to the bathroom. I had to call upon my mom for every little thing. The pain and the agony were unbelievable. I was not even able to move from side to side in bed. Every movement was monumental for me. I needed a great deal of physical help and thankfully, I got it. I was not able to work, exercise, socialize, or drive. I was the Walking Dead. I was very thin and weak. However, it was back to the hospital for me. I was getting really tired of it too. You know it is bad when the hospital staff recognizes you. The doctor had recommended a higher dosage of prednisone. The amount of Prednisone I was on, made me delirious. It is sad to say, and report that after 68 years of Lupus being discovered the only effective treatment for me was Prednisone. It is hard to believe, but true, there has not been a lot of research for Lupus patients and their families. It has only been in the past five years that they have come up with a new drug called Benlysta.

After my departure from the hospital, I had massive amounts of physical therapy. I worked for months and months on myself. I went three times a week and it was a grueling effort. I also went to many specialists for my feet, and they were not able to do anything for me. Deep down inside, I understood there was nothing that they could do for me. I was disheartened. The only way I knew I was going to be able to make a positive change in my life was motivating myself and building my self-esteem. As time moved on my self-confidence was slowly building. I did a great deal of spiritual healing and worked hard within myself by reading many books and listening to many tapes. It genuinely helped shape my way of thinking. Mind over matter, it is a very powerful tool. I do not think people realize how important a tool it really can be to assist you in your life.

I was working diligently and trying to get myself back slowly and than another set back. I had been working on my recovery for about two to two and half years. The cycle started again of not being able to walk, and my entire body started becoming inflamed. I really thought to myself, I could not go through this again. I ended up in the hospital, but this time my hospital visit was different. I had stayed for only three days. When they dismissed me, I had not fully recovered. It was because of the new health care laws. I was so angry, and weak. The reason for the early discharge was the hospital authorities felt there was nothing else they could do for me. I returned home extremely weak, my body still inflamed and filled with huge doses of Prednisone, I was beyond repair both physically and mentally. The doctors' had given me so many disgusting and nauseating addictive painkillers, and had increased my Cellcept,

Gabapentin, Prednisone, heart medication and God only knows what else... Despite all of this, I needed these medications to help me get back on track. Regardless of the crying and screaming that went on it would have been enough stress to kill someone. I was at my deepest depression for a couple of days, then I decided to have a talk with myself, and I said, "I can not have this negative mindset. I have to turn my life around and become me again." I remember the exact moment; I decided to move forward with my life. I thought long and hard about the implications, and the repercussions of what the rest of my life would be if I did not start to think positively. After that point, I decided to take total control of my life.

Once, I made my mind up to create a positive change and I would overcome my pain and agony. I decided to do some research on exercise, and I came up with a plan of action. I thought to myself and said, you have been an athlete your whole life, what sport could you do that would have no impact on your joints or cause you no bodily pain? The answer for me was swimming. First, I joined my local YMCA. The pool looked inviting and peaceful to me. I started by going once a week, and then twice a week, I slowly built up my stamina and endurance. I truly enjoyed swimming because it gave me a sense of harmony with myself. It allowed me to build my body one step at a time. The benefits that I got out it were priceless. I was able to start out in the pool by walking laps and doing water exercises to strengthen my core and my legs. In the beginning, I had not realized how weak my legs were and I was shocked. I decided to take one day at a time and not become overwhelmed.

I made a conscious effort every time I got into the pool to say my own positive mantras, which I made up myself. I was also thankful each day for what I had in my life. These positive thoughts helped shape me to become increasingly comfortable with myself and allowed me to strive for greater goals. As a result, I worked harder and my attitude was slowly changing for the better. My body was trying to come back and yet at the same time my DNA levels were still through the roof. This meant my inflammation was still running high throughout my body. My Rheumatologist had several attempts and conversations with me to try this new drug called Benlysta. I was acutely resistant with good cause, because of what happened to me with the Chemo. I just could not take another bad side effect, which would leave me with permanent damage. I was working hard trying to take control of mind and body that I did not want any more wrenches thrown at me. I was a smart cookie because I told the doctor let's wait and see how the other patients do on the new Benlysta. I wanted to see if there were any detrimental side effects from this new drug. I waited a little over a year until I decided to conform to the doctor, and try the Benlysta. I told him, "I would only try it, if I could do the medicine month by month, and I would stop it if I felt or saw anything going awry with my body." He agreed to my request. My outcome for the very first time that I have had Lupus was a positive one and benefited me greatly. I could not believe it! God was finally listening to my prayers and I was on my way to a new path in my life. Looking back, I always wanted to be a Psychiatrist. However, in high school, I was in Chemistry class and I fainted at the sight of my own blood. I fell onto my face and chipped all of my four front teeth. My Dad had to come to school and he literally picked me up off the floor. As I awoke, I remember thinking that I was just finishing up on a roller coaster ride.

My Dad came and got me because his dental office was literally three minutes from my high school and the nuns knew him well. He capped my teeth and the rest is history. Therefore, I never chose to be a doctor. However, the irony in my life is that I would always have to be giving blood and having it taken for lab testing. I quickly got over the fear of fainting because I always had my blood taken on a consistent basis. I wish I had become a doctor, because I would have been an amazing one.

Chapter 6

Slow Change

"When I loved myself enough, I began leaving whatever wasn't healthy. This meant people, jobs, and my own beliefs and habits and anything that I thought made me small. My judgment called it disloyal. I see it as self-loving."

Kim McMiller

My Benlysta, infusions were working slowly and my immune system was trying to regulate itself. My DNA levels were starting to drop. According to my doctor, they were no longer off the charts. He was pleased, as was I, with the results. It has been a slow process, but a good one for me both physically and mentally. A few months after my infusions, I started to have more energy and I could feel the inflammation in my body decreasing. This was all positive news, but the best news of all was I was not having any severe side effects from the medication, as I had had from the Chemo. My mind was at ease and for the first time in sixteen years, I had felt a little sliver of freedom from my illness. As I gained more self–confidence within myself, I was feeling better and being able to move more freely. My outlook on my future took a turn for the better. I knew I could do anything that I wanted to do with my life and not live in fear. However, for the last 20 years, I have lived in fear of what my life would be and how I was going to live it. Now, I can honestly say, no more. I do not live my life in fear, but in strength. It has become my mantra on a daily basis. It is hard to stick with it everyday, but I keep trying. It seems to be working for me as long as I keep a positive attitude. I would be lying if I said; "I am happy everyday and every moment of my life." Nobody on this planet lives his or her life in that way. Reality is the best way to deal with your life. If you can look into the mirror everyday and be grateful for what you have then you have accomplished a lot. I can honestly say, I look in the mirror everyday and count my blessings. I make sure that I give a big smile to myself and I smile back to the universe.

As I gradually started to feel like a real person again, I started to make small changes in my diet and exercise. I had been to many nutritionists over the years and had learned about many different ways to handle my dietary needs. However, I had to find my own gratified way to make my body harmonious with proper nutrition for me. It has made a world of difference to me both physically and mentally. The saying, "you are what you eat" is true. I believe and have experienced when I eat a well and balanced diet my results are I am a well-balanced individual. It allows me to be productive and to have a positive attitude to take on the world each day.

In the past, my diet was unhealthy for me. I would eat many fried and processed foods. I would drink many sugary drinks including soda. All of these things were detrimental to my body. It caused me to have great inflammation with my body's immune system. I cannot explain the pain that certain types of foods would give me that would cause my hands, knees and feet to become inflamed. There were times when I could not bend my fingers or bend my knees properly let alone to have my feet swollen. Food is so essential in order to have good health. I learned the hard way, by trail and error. I found that I am allergic to certain foods and if I eat them, they are not good for me. My body does not respond well. As for my diet, I eat a lot of protein; vegetables, fruit and I drink water all the time. It cleans out your system and it is excellent for your complexion.

In general, for me, my body does not respond well to medications. No two people who have Lupus have the same exact type of symptoms of having the disease. What works for me might not work for someone else who has Lupus. It makes sense because everyone's immune system is different when dealing with a disease. The way that I work my nutrition now is whatever I put into my body; it should come out of me naturally. I have given up salt and garlic. I use to love the both of them, but they cause me inflammation in my body. I use to also eat a lot of tomato sauce. I can only have organic or real homemade Italian sauce from a specialty store. I think because the other sauces are processed and filled with a high amount of salt and sugar. I have given up soda and I have never been a coffee drinker. I try to avoid caffeine. I have been cutting back on bread and food with nitrates. I love chicken so much; I think I could turn into a chicken. I eat it almost everyday. I eat red meat once a week. It is just that I am not a big fan of the taste of red meat. I eat oatmeal and I drink milk everyday. Milk is a very important part of my diet especially as a woman. I need calcium and Vitamin D. I was smart enough to have it on a daily basis because if I did not over the last 18 years, while I was on Prednisone, I would have severe bone loss. The result of taking Prednisone for last 18 years caused me bone loss and has weakened my bones. Luckily, I only have Osteopenia, which is about 2% bone loss in my body, and I am grateful everyday that I only have that amount of loss.

As for my teeth, I have completely given up gum. One summer, I decided to chew gum to help curb my appetite. I just wanted to try to lose a lit bit of extra weight. I scheduled my dental appointment, and I find out that I needed to have three root canals done on my upper left part of my mouth, Unbelievable! The medications over the years have destroyed both my gums and teeth. Think about it, your immune system connects to every part of your body. I have dental cleanings every three months. I have worked hard on taking care of my teeth as a result, my teeth look good and I been blessed with a gorgeous smile! I believe that your smile is everything. You can change a persons' day just by smiling at them and they smile back at you. It is important for me to take care of my mouth, since my father was a dentist. When I was a teenager, I use to work in his office on a Saturday. I enjoyed it and learned a lot about teeth. My diet affects my teeth and I carefully watch the type of food and drink that I eat. I have found the things I do for myself regarding my dental care have really helped me maintain good dental hygiene.

Over time, I have been able to find balance between my mind and body connection. I try to categorize the issues that I have physically with my Lupus and then categorize the issues that I have mentally with my Lupus. Then, I try to mesh them together in a way that my body can be in harmony. It has taken me many years to accomplish this goal in my life. The following things that I need to accomplish my daily goals are exercise, meditation, reading, writing, reducing and maintaining stress levels, eating well, sleeping well and finally keeping hydrated with lots of water. It is essential that I keep this routine. I take my medications at the same time everyday which helps regulate my body to have a better and blessed day.

I work within my parameters that fit into my lifestyle. It is hard to face the music in your life when you have had to make so many life changes. I have learned to transform the things in my life that are not beneficial for me my job, friendships and personal relationships. I had many conversions about them because I have had a lot of transition with my personality and my personal needs. It is not a big deal or negative in your life if you have to let go of certain friends or relationships. I truly believe that if things do not work out, then it was not supposed to be, and it is for the better. I believe in fate, especially since I have been through all of these experiences over the last 20 years of my life. I have learned many things since I have had my Lupus. I believe with great conviction that it is my calling to help people who do have it and to inspire them to continue with their lives in a positive way.

Chapter 7

Determination

"It's not whether you get knocked down, it's whether you get up."

Vince Lombardi

Yoga, stretching, core building, cardio, swimming, and walking are all different types of exercises that are helpful in making your body feel good and build strength. There are no excuses to want to build your body, mind, and soul up to be happy. It takes discipline, determination and perseverance. I believe that anyone can do it. You have to be hungry for it, like a wolf. You have to want to do it and you have to want to overcome whatever is ailing you inside of your body. You must say to yourself, "I can do this, I am strong, beautiful, happy, powerful, all knowing and I love myself." If you love yourself, you will be motivated to just do it.

It is important for me to do some type of exercise on a daily basis. It allows me to have a sense of freedom, which in turn gives me positivity and allows me to execute my goals for the day. I have done various exercises over the years to get me started with building my body strong. I know and realize that money is a factor when you have an illness. The physical activities that I have done over the years do not cost a lot of money. Joining a gym or your local YMCA is beneficial. It allows you to have access to many activities for the price of a monthly fee or yearly membership. I have taken yoga classes and they are wonderful for both my mind and body. If you start out with one class and build yourself up to, what you want to achieve. I love them because they make me feel good. Everyday, I stretch and do breathing exercises. Stretching invigorates the body. Posture is important. You always want to stand tall and proud. Image is everything. I believe you always have to look good no matter what is going on in your life. Take pride in yourself. It helps you to feel better about yourself.

After starting to exercise and strengthening my core, it has granted me to have more self-confidence and self-esteem within myself. Myself image has flourished and now everyday, when I wake up I feel like I am putting on my suit of armor. I am ready to step out into the world in a confident way. It all starts with baby steps, taking your time and going by your own rhythm. I believe that it has to only come from within you and nobody else.

Cardio and swimming have really helped me with my endurance. I use to have zero endurance and now I have an abundance of it. When you have SLE Lupus heart issues come into play. Unfortunately, for me and I'm assuming a lot of other people who have Lupus, high blood pressure is a staple when you're taking lots of medications. I had high blood pressure for 18 years. I had a hard time with it a few years ago. I had to go to the hospital for it and I was scared. I kept thinking, am I going to I have a heart attack? It took me a while, but I got it back under control. The cardiologist has also told me that by having the high blood pressure it does take a toll on your heart, as you get older. Lupus affects your major organs in your body.

Walking and moving all the time is great for anyone. It helps you clear your mind and it keeps you active. Busy is a good thing. The more positive thoughts you can create for yourself the more you will want to do and achieve. Perception is everything. I am an avid reader of self-help, spiritual, financial, photography, autobiographies and history books. I listen to many self-healing and spiritual tapes while I am driving the car. It allows me to focus on me. It took me many years to learn that I come first in my life. I am a giver not a taker. I have had to learn to give myself permission to be selfish in a gratifying way. I am still a giver. I just put my health first now, before I do anything else. I am proud to have learned this lesson.

Advocacy is a crucial ingredient in taking care of yourself when you have Lupus. I have always been and will be my best advocate. It's key to know your patient's, "Bill of Rights" when you are a patient in a hospital. Remember, the doctor and/or doctors are not God. They do not have all the answers to heal you. You may want to ask questions. It is helpful if you have a list for the doctor. If your not able to then you need to designate someone close to you to be your advocate.

My experience has lead me to believe that it doesn't matter how good or bad the hospital is or the care that you're receiving you need to always keep on top of the situation. I have always kept a notebook, a folder and complete medical records each time I have had a hospital stay. I have learned to trust my instincts and always listen to what my body is telling me. I believe that each individual knows what is best for him or her. I advise anyone to always listen when the doctor speaks to you about your illness. Try to learn as much as possible and have a good comprehension of it. It is always good to be able to have a well-educated conversation with a medical professional, when you are proficient about your Lupus or any illness you may have.

I have had many mishaps with my health care, and yes, it has maddened me. However, I have always taken the high road and have followed the proverb by Elbert Hubbard, "When life gives you lemons, make lemonade." Initially, I am always distraught and frustrated, but then I calm down and try to look at my situation in a positive light. There are always two sides to situations in life. I have learned to choose the side that benefits me. Actually, since having my Lupus I have become a good problem solver. It has allowed me to look and create more than one option when something negative turns up in my life. I feel blessed that I have developed this character trait about myself. It has become a good tool for me to have in my hat. It has become easier for me to make good decisions for myself.

I have always believed in education. "Knowledge is power." The more knowledge that I have the more powerful I am. I am a lifetime learner. I love to learn about anything, especially the things in my life that I am passionate about learning. Learn as much as you possibly can, it cannot hurt you. It can only help you. I think that another key tool to have in one's hat is attitude. I have the attitude that I am always a kid inside myself. I believe if you keep the mindset of being childlike, adventurous, free spirited and having fun it will carry you through life in a magical way. Do not allow anyone to belittle you or tell you no, in your life. Do not believe it. Believe in yourself and your dreams. If you have no dreams, you are dying inside, but if you have dreams, you are living your life and trying to strive to be or do something great for yourself. My attitude has always been to persevere. I believe I can do and be anything I put my mind to do. By having much faith, knowledge and understanding about life, it has helped me accomplish my goals and dreams.

There are many challenges to face when confronted with an illness. I believe there is two ways to face your challenge, either accept it head on or reject it and lay down. I have always chosen to accept my challenge. It is hard to look into the mirror everyday and see your reality. However, it is best to accept it and move forward with your life. It is not easy to do because there are so many factors surrounding a person who is dealing with an illness. I have found being organized has helped me tremendously. I organize myself on a daily basis. I make lists of things that I must do and another list for things I would like to do. My work schedule, finances, medical reports/papers, exercise, diet, social life are all in order. This allows me to be productive and positive. I use my iPhone calendar to help get organized and I keep a paper calendar for my work. I write daily for both personal and professional reasons. Time management is another key element in helping when facing a challenge. Stress is a huge factor when you have Lupus. I try to minimize my stress levels by controlling the things that I am able to control and I let go of the things that I cannot control. This has taken me many years to learn and I am still learning. As time goes on, I have better time management skills and organizational skills, which allow me to have a better mental focus and reduce my stress levels.

Over the years with my Lupus, I use to take in my stress and in turn, internalize it. It was detrimental to my health. I would become physically sick and my body would become inflamed with pain in my joints. I would have zero energy and I was extremely fatigued all the time. This was one of the hardest things that I had to learn to help control my Lupus. It was key for me. I am a type "A" person, which most Lupus patients are and I have learned to take a step back. It is important to analyze the situation and not make rash decisions. I have made many rash decisions due to the types of medications that I have taken especially having been on the prednisone. Prednisone would make me agitated, aggressive, irritable, moody and depressed. I knew that all of these things were going on with me. I had to figure out how to minimize the side effects. I found two things that helped me reduce these side effects, water and exercise. Water cleanses the body and exercise reduces inflammation in your body. I have been to the best of the best doctors and have gone to holistic doctors. I have tried many natural remedies too. I found that water and exercise have helped me control my Lupus.

Doctors' diagnosis and the treatment of diseases and conditions come in many forms including medication, procedures, surgery or therapy. Doctors can treat your symptoms, but the individual has to want to heal oneself. I believe that mind over matter comes into play when trying to battle a disease. This is exactly what happened to me in dealing with my disease. Twenty years ago, my first rheumatologist stated to me that I would not be able to move my hands and fingers on a permanent basis. Moreover, I would not live a good life. My life expectancy was unknown. It felt like a Mac Truck was hitting me. It was beyond words combined with great anger. I knew that I would survive this disease. It almost got me a few times, but I had the will and the power to survive. I am here to tell you that you can become a survivor too!

We all fall, but it is our own decision on whether or not we want to get back up and try again. I am here to tell you "Lupus is only a word, not a label." Make something of yourself that brings you joy and happiness. Life is too short, celebrate the little moments and try to make yourself special again. Society does not know much about Lupus. I have always felt like it is a dirty disease. No one knows what it is or how to try to deal with it. According to current statistics, Lupus affects women by 90% and men by 10%. It is primarily a women's disease. Approximately 70% of all accounts of Lupus are Systemic Lupus. It develops in people at the ages of 15 to 44. Education and research are key elements to helping us with this disease. I have made it my mission to let people know and to have a better understanding of the disease. I have never seen a celebrity as a spokesperson for Lupus. I would like to take Lupus to the forefront and empower women who have the disease. It is important for them to know they have support and education to help them to have a better life. Lupus has no boundaries.

I have written to many celebrities who have Lupus and have never received an answer. I figured at some point someone would answer me. My mission now is to make Lupus as well known as other diseases like Heart disease, Diabetes, Cancer, AIDs, etc. It is important that our disease gets recognition. The more people who know about it the more money will go towards research for developing new drugs, which are in desperate need. There are only a handful of drugs to treat Lupus. I believe that more public service announcements about Lupus on social media will bring more recognition for the disease. The good news is that the major Lupus Foundations are forming into one large foundation concerning Lupus. This is an excellent idea of joining forces and resources together to make a positive impact on Lupus.

After my sister passed in 1989, I decided to set up a fund in honor of her name with the Long Island Community Foundation and the fund is The Ann Caroline Corredy Fund. Every year, for the last 16 years, I have given money to a Lupus organizations' primarily for research. In the past, I have given money to Camp Sunshine, which allows families with Lupus to spend a designated week in Maine during the summer. Three years ago, I volunteered for the Lupus week with their families. It was an unforgettable experience. I have also written a children's story for the SLE Foundation in New York. I have donated monies to the SLE Foundation in New York, Lupus Alliance of Long Island Queens, and Alliance for Lupus Research. I have participated in Lupus walks and 5K's. In addition, I have an article about me concerning my Lupus in the issue of Web MD for October 2014 for Lupus Awareness Month. I believe that Christopher Reeve said it best, "Success is finding satisfaction in giving a little more than you take."

Chapter 8

Balance

"When you love and accept yourself, when you know who really cares about you, and when you learn from your mistakes, then you stop caring about what people who don't know you think."

Beyoncé Knowles

I believe the most important factor in handling an illness is caring for oneself. You need to be self-serving. It is the most challenging factor to deal with in the healing process. You must follow your own path with courage and kindness. It is very difficult to deal with a deck of cards that you been dealt, and have no choice, but to change. I know and understand that transformation is hard, but it is the pathway to healing and becoming healthy again. Everyone wants to feel well. It is only natural. Particularly for me, I call it feeling normal.

Change waltzed into my life like a dance. For the last twenty years, each day and year has been a challenge for me whether I liked it or not. It has been immensely difficult. It has invoked fear and fear has implored uncertainty and loss. Metamorphosis with an illness conjures up the thought of having more pain than you already have or have been through. I remember every time, I had a medical test or been given new medications I would be alarmed. It was the uncertainty that would stress me out. It was the lack of control, I had over my physical body and it was difficult to deal with. However, the one thing I have learned over the years is that I can control my mental state along with my emotions. It has been a long hard journey to get to where I am today, mentally. Your mental state of mind is key when dealing with change.

Many factors come into play when dealing with change. For me it was my expectations and the process of what was going to happen to me next with my illness, it was constantly changing. I had to alter my focus on myself and accept the transformation. I decided to learn and grow from it, which helped me heal myself.

Change is either positive or negative. I choose it to be positive. I had to be self-serving to myself with all my hospitalizations, tests, new medications and handling my emotional state. I always have to handle change. It has become a staple in my life. Most people have to handle change on a small scale, but for me it has been like a colossal roller coaster, up and down. My body and mind are always transitioning depending upon the status of my health. The one thing about me is that I am too positive to be doubtful. I work through the things and issues that confront me.

Drive in my life has helped me to bring about change in order for me to heal myself. I have drive everyday to become stronger and smarter about myself. Setting goals and facing my challenges helps me achieve my transition in a positive light. I try to focus heavily each day with what I want to accomplish. I want to engage and energize myself with a positive attitude, which leads to good health. Remember, without your health, you have nothing in life. I know this because I have been there and done that and it was the darkest point in my journey. When you do not have health, it is difficult to have your basic needs met. This is where your life turns on you and it feels like you are spinning out of control. It is always important to have balance. Everyone has to find his or her own balance or I call it formula that works for them. Harmony is necessary to achieve balance in your life. There are many ways of finding harmony. As I have stated previously that Lupus affects each individual differently, therefore a person's definition of harmony is going to be different for everyone. It is very individualized. I cannot give you an exact plan or formula. I can only explain to you what has worked for me. Resources and tools have helped me a great deal in my healing process.

I believe that "God gives you the face that you deserve." God has given me a lovely face considering all the things that I have been through with my scares, burns and trauma with my Lupus. Sometimes, I look at myself and I do not understand why I look the way I do. I could have had a very bad outcome with my skin and I have been very blessed. It is important to put gratefulness out into the universe on a daily basis.

My Balance Formula

The traits listed below have helped me build myself. In a metaphorical way, they assist me to wear my "hat" everyday. I call them pins. (The pins are not in any specific order.) I have no responsibility for your outcome, as I am not a medical professional.

Pin# 1- Attitude

Pin# 2- Self-Serving

Pin# 3- Gratitude

Pin# 4- Exercise

Pin# 5- Outlook

Pin# 6- Spirituality

Pin# 7- Self-Confidence

Pin# 8- Self–Esteem

Pin# 9- Learning and Knowledge

Pin# 10- Accepting Change

Pin# 11- Sleep

Pin# 12- Writing

Pin# 13- Advocacy

Pin# 14- Charity

Pin# 15- Organization

Pin# 16- Therapy-Physical and Mental

Pin# 17- Drive

Pin# 18- Perseverance

Pin# 19- Motivation

Pin# 20- Relaxation

Pin# 21- Mediation

Pin# 22- Harmony

Pin# 23- Peace

Pin# 24- Honesty

Pin# 25- Faith

Pin# 26- Dreams

Pin#27- Discipline

Pin# 28- Listening

Pin# 29- Commitment

Pin# 30- A Big Smile

These pins have granted me to be present, more patient, and to stay on task, which has led me to become more goal oriented. They let me acquiesce my own focus on a daily basis and they have given me the gift of life. I can truly say that I am living again as "me." I have worked tirelessly on myself and it has paid off. It takes a lot to pick yourself up and put yourself back together. In the beginning of my journey the analogy, that I liked to use was I was a "broken doll" who needed to be mended. Now, I am proud to say that I have done an awesome job of mending myself back to a "beautiful doll."

It has taken me years to be the woman who I am. My life has been irrevocable, closed, presently it belongs to me, and therefore, I am. When you put positive intentions out into the universe it will allow you to attract what you want to come into your life. All of my pins that I wear in my "hat" have taught me to have a full life.

Chapter 9

I've Risen to the Occasion

"With a new day comes new strength and new thoughts."

Eleanor Roosevelt

Currently, I am no longer on my Benlysta infusions, my neuropathy has worsened in my feet and I still have a problem in my right eye. However, I try not to become discouraged with the changes in my body. I just work with a positive outlook and attitude everyday. I am strong and I am whole. My body and mind will stay connected to deal with my physical changes. I have my Balance Formula and I will use it wisely. I have gained a lot of knowledge and have learned how to process the changes in my life. I believe that I have this gift of helping others who are trying to heal themselves with a disease.

I use a self-motivating checklist, which allows me to choose which step I want to reach on a daily basis. I have two methods of using it, writing it down or doing a mental checklist in my head. It is a great action tool. I acquired it while I was substitute teaching at an elementary school. The author is unknown. It consists of eight steps. You can apply it to anything you are trying to achieve on your health journey towards healing.

Here are the steps:

Step 1- I won't do it, or

Step 2- I can't do it, or

Step 3- I want to do it, or

Step 4- How do I do it? or

Step 5- I'll try to do it, or

Step 6- I can do it, or

Step 7- I will do it, or

Step 8- YES, I DID IT!

It is easy, you choose your own level of comfort and it is very individualized. There is no right or wrong answer on how to handle what you choose to do.

I am an author, wellness activist and Lupus survivor. I believe that I will be able to inspire others and help them on their journeys. I believe in giving back, and at the same time, it gives me great satisfaction. It is a win, win situation for all. If anyone would like to contact me, my email address is aimeeackell@gmail.com or you can visit my website at www.aimeeackell.com I would welcome the opportunity to do a motivational presentation to help individuals in their daily lives.

I would love to speak at the following Venues:

Bookstores

Churches

Clinics

Corporations

Business Clubs and Groups

Hospitals

Synagogues

Trade Shows

Health Clubs and Sport's Teams

Beauty Spas

Schools and Colleges

Women's Interest Groups and Associations

Special Groups and Organizations

Youth Organizations and Clubs

Public Libraries

My Educational background entails an undergraduate degree from George Washington University in D.C. with a B.A. in Economics. I attended, Teacher's Institute at Oxford University, Oxford, England. I hold two Masters degrees from Adelphi University, Garden City, New York, with an M.A. in Elementary and Physical Education and my second M.S. from Long Island University, C.W. Post College, Brookville, NY with an M.S.L.I.S., Master's in Library Information Science.

While I was walking on my own path, I believe that I saw my own purpose. As you walk through your journey, you learn from it, and your purpose is right in front of you. It is important to listen, learn and laugh at yourself. You can remove the distractions from your environment, but do not pull entirely away from everything in your world.

By realizing my true potential, I am ready for the life that I am destined to live. I treat myself how I would like to be treated. I believe that we all need to stay strong, focus on the "light" and be gracious towards others. I have gone through a lot in my life and not to compare it to what my sister experienced. I am just an individual bringing awareness to the forefront about Lupus. I believe in education, and continuing education. You can never have too much of it. I am a strong woman who can be gentle, I am educated, but humble, I am fierce, but compassionate, and I have discipline, therefore I can be free.

In the past, I use to feel this way when I spoke to people and I was not able to tell them about my life with my Lupus. I wrote this poem called "Mask."

Mask

I wear a Mask everyday

Hiding, and wanting to scream inside, "I'm Ok"

However, people do not see me that way

They say "Oh you look great"

"You're so beautiful"

If they only knew the truth, the pain and the hurt inside

I feel like I cannot be myself all the time, cause they don't understand

Me

I wear a Mask everyday

I have had to give up everything and make serious life changes

I am not the same person that I use to be

I wish, I was normal, back to my original self

I do not think the time will ever come again

New times, new life and a new Mask for everyday

So sad, that I have to hide behind my Mask

I wish, I didn't have to wear my Mask and be judged everyday

I just want myself back, and no more Mask

I wrote this on October 17, 2011. I had no idea that I would be where I am today. I have come such a long way through my journey and the result is I did get myself back and I do not have to wear a "Mask" anymore. I believe subconsciously that I willed myself to take off my "Mask" and to show the world, who I really am. I am a young vibrant, beautiful, intelligent, adventurous, loving, giving, enthusiastic, hard-working and self-confident woman emerging from her cocoon.

I found this quote from Living Color (www.Laughthecolors.com)

No one has the perfect life, which begins with "Once upon a time" and ends with "Happily ever after."

"Life begins with a welcome to the struggle and ends with you are lucky to have survived the journey.

If you wait for happy moments, you will wait forever….

But if you start believing that, you are happy

You will be happy forever…

Remember all the problems are stuck between the Mind and Matter.

If you don't Mind,

It does not Matter."

I believe this sums it all up about life and one's journey. I am very proud of myself to have shared my story with all of you. I hope you have enjoyed reading it and it has delivered a powerful and positive message.

Chapter 10

Thankfulness

"Gratitude is the key that unlocks every door."

Unknown

I have always been grateful for what I have, and for what I have done in my life. Gratitude has unlocked many doors for me. I believe whatever you put into the universe you get back in your life. There is nothing wrong with being a gracious person who behaves with courage, kindness, compassion, respect and dignity. The motto that I have lived by is always being kind, gracious, giving, and loving toward others.

I would like to say thank you to the following people who have helped me along the way on my Lupus Journey. The first groups of people I want to thank are my doctors. Thanks to Dr. Gerald Appel affiliated with New York-Presbyterian Hospital for taking care of my kidneys. You are an awesome doctor and diagnostician.

Dr. Philip Ragone affiliated with St. Francis Hospital thanks for taking care of me neurologically. I truly appreciate your kindness and support throughout the years. You are the best!

Dr. Jules Garbus, MD my kind colon and rectal man, who handled me with delicate care.

Dr. Andrew Porges and his staff affiliated with NYU-Langone, Rheumatology Associates-Long Island. Many thanks for all the wonderful care and support you have given me. I believe that out of all of my doctors, you have seen the most growth overall in my health.

Dr. Brian Cooperman affiliated with Northern Obstetrics & Gynecology, I truly love and respect you so much as my Gynecologist. You have helped me through so many trying times throughout my Lupus journey. I am forever grateful. You are amazing at what you do and how you treat your patients. We have had many talks and discussions about life. You have always given me sound advice. You are very special to me.

Dr. Tharakaram Ravishankar my Internist, I have known you the longest out of all my doctors and you have helped me out tremendously. I am grateful to you for your years of service and care that you have given to me.

Dr. Joseph Minadeo affiliated with St. Francis Hospital you have been a great Cardiologist, and you have taken excellent care of my heart. I am grateful that my heart has not skipped a beat.

Dr. Lawrence Ostroff, DPM affiliated with Kotkin & Ostroff you have been a blessing to me for my feet. I have had so many issues with them, and you have cared for them, oh so delicately. I know that I am safe with you and you always put me back on my feet.

Dr. Bruce Goldman, DDS you have made my smile brighter. People tell me, "What a lovely smile, I have." I am happy to have found you to help me with my dental care. You always do fantastic job on my teeth.

Dr. Robert C. Ferris, DDS, my Orthodontist, thanks for helping me keep my pearly white teeth in alignment. I always wear my retainer. You are always so kind and gentle when working in my mouth.

Dr. Raymond L. Soletic, MD I am lucky to have found such a nice Ear, Nose and Throat doctor. Your level of care and attention to detail is outstanding in helping me with many of my medical issues.

Last, but no least Dr. John P. Brennan and Dr. D'Arienzo for helping me with my eyes. I believe that my eyes show and tell who I am. Without my vision, I would not be able to see.

I would like to give heartfelt thanks and blessings to all of my family members who have helped me throughout the years. I am thankful to all my brothers for there help and support. Mark, Paul, Edward and Thomas. You all have inspired me to do well for myself and work hard.

My sister, Christine thanks for all your assistance over the years. You have always been there for me and I especially want to thank my other sister "Ann" was has passed on from this disease. Your memory of love and laughter will always live on.

To all of my extend family, my in-laws: Boyd, Cindy, and Laura thanks for everything that you have done for me. I appreciate it. Thanks to my nieces and nephews and their wives too. Brandon, Melissa, Makayla,

Olivia and Samantha. Stephen, Rebecca, Avery and Bradleigh. Bryon, Kelly and Mackenzie. Eric, Bryttannee and Aryk. Matthew, Christian, Emily Ann, Natalie, Maximus, James and Lucas you have always cheered me up in my times of my sickness.

I cannot say thank you enough to my Mom for doing all things that you have done for me. "Mother, I love you!"

Thanks to all of my friends who have done so many things for me over the years. We have all listened and laughed together through the good and the bad times. "Merci Beaucoup"- to Stevie Cianciulli, Wanda Wilken, Leonard Ogbonna, Christine Boryk, Josiane Peluso, Diane Hanna, Donna Hanna, Catherine Vidal, Lois Tubby, Steve Russell Boerner, Margaret Ippolito, Nina Glenn, Cynthia Dano, The Forman family, Jimmy and Ann Wood, Tony and Rose Gallo, Rose Laurie, Ginnie Paniccia, Karen Puritano, Lynn Scarpati, William Tanzi, Eric Saretsky, Sal and Florence Anselmo, Nancy Lan, and William Petrusky.

"Grazie"- to all of my gym friends who have inspired me to be the best that I can be physically. I enjoy all of you on a daily basis. Especially, Alex Bonis, Ed Marinello, Stan Pitera, Bryant Dorman and Kristen Lee Taylor, you are like family to me.

"Gracias"- to Julio Almonte for helping me create and complete my beautiful web site and to Mike Swedenberg for helping me edit my story.

"Happiness- Gratitude and peace with the past + full engagement in the present + enthusiasm for tomorrow." –Brenden Burchard-

I think this quote sums up all my gratitude toward everyone in my life, past and present. I will leave you with these two final quotes that I found and I believe to be true.

"You're braver than you believe and stronger than you seem, and smarter than you think." -Christopher Robin-

I have found that to be true for myself on the journey that I have been on and will continue. I do not know what my life brings me next, but I believe that I will receive an abundance of great blessings.

"Learn to love without condition. Talk without bad intention. Give without any reason. And most of all, care for people without any expectation." –Quote of the Day-

This quote is very inspiring to me and I intend to keep it close to my heart while on my "Butterfly Girl," My Lupus Journey. As I have said before my greatest pleasure in my life is that when people tell me "I can't, I turn around, and say, I can!"

My final realization, as I sat in church on a Sunday, and I looked up at the high ceiling and saw the word "Pax" which means "peace." I realized what my Lupus journey had meant to me. I had found my true meaning of health and happiness, it's a combination of "Peace + Harmony." I hope that my message has helped you and you can walk along your journey in peace and harmony.

ABOUT THE AUTHOR

Aimee Ackell is an author, motivational speaker and wellness activist. In 2010, her revelation and wake-up moment have allowed her to make a lifestyle change with her health. This has allowed her to empower herself and others who are Lupus warriors. Her remarkable journey has led her to diminish the stress factors and increase the "Aha Moments" which life has to offer. Throughout her journey, nature and spirituality have encouraged her spirit daily.

Aimee Ackell is the founder of her sister's fund, The Ann Caroline Corredy Fund through The Long Island Community Foundation. She donates monies every year to various Lupus organizations for research in hope for a cure for Lupus and other autoimmune diseases. She hopes for a bright future for everyone. She resides in Glen Head, New York.

Made in the USA
Middletown, DE
29 April 2016